Rapamycin and Lifespan Extension

A very short introduction from
The HealthSpan Institute

Rapamycin and Lifespan Extension
A Very Short Introduction from The HealthSpan Institute

ISBN: 9798865012221

Printed in the United States of America

Contents

Chapter 1:
Introduction

Chapter 2:
Background on Rapamycin

Chapter 3:
Rapamycin and Aging:
The Research Journey

Chapter 4:
Potential Mechanisms:
How Does Rapamycin Influence Aging?

Chapter 5:
Challenges and Controversies

Chapter 6:
Broader Impacts of Rapamycin on Health

Chapter 7:
Future of Rapamycin and Lifespan Extension

Chapter 8:
Conclusions

Appendix A:
Glossary of Terms

Appendix B:
Detailed Results from Key Studies

Appendix C:
Resources for Further Reading and Exploration

References

Chapter 1: Introduction

Brief History of Lifespan Research

From the time humans first began to understand their own mortality, there has been an innate curiosity about the boundaries of life and the possibility of extending its duration. Lifespan research has a rich and storied history that bridges ancient practices, philosophical inquiries, and modern scientific investigations.

Ancient Civilizations and the Quest for Immortality

Historical records indicate that ancient civilizations, from the Sumerians to the Egyptians and the Chinese, held deep fascinations with immortality and youth. Elixirs, rituals, and myths were centered around the pursuit of life extension. The famous tale of the "Elixir of Life" in Chinese mythology, or the story of the philosopher's stone in Western alchemical tradition, are testaments to humanity's age-old desire to conquer death.

The Middle Ages and Renaissance: Alchemy and Early Medicine

During the Middle Ages, alchemists across Europe sought substances that could transform base metals into gold, cure all diseases, and grant eternal life. While their pursuits often blended mysticism with proto-science, they laid the foundation for modern chemistry and medicine. The Renaissance period saw a burgeoning interest in the human body, anatomy, and the nature of life and death. Scientists and thinkers like Leonardo da Vinci began to study the human body with greater rigor, setting the stage for future investigations into human health and longevity.

The Enlightenment: The Dawn of Modern Biology

The Enlightenment brought about a methodical, empirical approach to science. As researchers began to categorize and understand the natural world, the study of biology and the human lifespan became a distinct field of inquiry. It was during this period that scientists began to look at lifespan not just as a fixed trait, but as something that could be influenced by external factors, like diet and environment.

The 20th Century: Genetics and Molecular Biology

The discovery of the DNA double helix in the 1950s was a turning point in lifespan research. With the understanding of genetics, researchers began to unravel the mysteries of aging at a molecular level. The latter half of the century saw breakthroughs in the understanding of cellular aging, the role of telomeres, and the mechanics of genetic inheritance which all have implications for lifespan. Studies on model organisms, from yeast to fruit flies and mice, have provided insights into genes and pathways that influence aging and longevity.

Modern Era: Integrating Biotechnology and AI

The late 20th and early 21st centuries heralded the era of biotechnology. With the mapping of the human genome and advancements in technologies like CRISPR for gene editing, there was a renewed hope for understanding the genetic underpinnings of aging and potentially intervening in the aging process. Furthermore, with the rise of artificial intelligence and big data analytics, researchers can now analyze vast amounts of information, accelerating discoveries in lifespan extension.

In recent decades, the focus of lifespan research has shifted subtly from simply extending life to enhancing the quality of those additional years, termed 'healthspan'. This recognizes the importance of not just living longer, but living better. The discovery of compounds like rapamycin, which seem to influence the aging process itself, is a testament to how far the field has come.

In conclusion, the history of lifespan research is a tapestry of human curiosity, interwoven with myths, early scientific inquiries, and groundbreaking modern discoveries. From the ancients' quest for immortality to today's cutting-edge labs, the journey of understanding and potentially extending the human lifespan is a narrative of human tenacity, hope, and relentless inquiry.

Introduction to Rapamycin and Its Discovery

Rapamycin, a compound that has generated considerable excitement in the world of lifespan research, stands out not only for its potential anti-aging properties but also for its intriguing origin story. Its journey from a remote island to the forefront of scientific investigation is both serendipitous and emblematic of the unpredictable nature of discovery in the world of biomedicine.

Origins: From Easter Island to the Laboratory

Rapamycin's tale begins on the remote Easter Island, known locally as Rapa Nui, situated in the southeastern Pacific Ocean. In 1964, a team of Canadian scientists journeyed to this isolated location, known for its mysterious stone statues, on an expedition to collect soil samples. The goal was simple: to explore novel microbial life in diverse environments, with the hope of uncovering substances with potential therapeutic benefits.

It was within these soil samples that researchers discovered a unique bacterium, *Streptomyces hygroscopicus*. This bacterium produced a compound that demonstrated potent antifungal activity. Named "rapamycin" after the island of its discovery, initial interest in the compound revolved around its potential as an antifungal agent. However, subsequent research would unveil its far-reaching implications in medicine and biology.

Unveiling Rapamycin's Medical Potential

The initial excitement surrounding rapamycin as an antifungal agent waned as researchers identified its potent immunosuppressive properties. This unexpected discovery shifted the focus of rapamycin's potential applications. By the 1980s and 1990s, rapamycin began to be explored as a possible drug to prevent organ transplant rejection due to its ability to suppress the immune system.

The molecular target of rapamycin was identified in the early 1990s, furthering the understanding of its mechanism of action. This target, a protein aptly named the "mechanistic target of rapamycin" or mTOR, plays a central role in regulating cell growth, proliferation, and survival. It was this interaction with the mTOR pathway that hinted at rapamycin's broader implications, not just in transplantation medicine, but in cancer, metabolism, and eventually, aging.

The Aging Connection

The turning point for rapamycin in the context of lifespan research came when scientists began to investigate its effects on the aging process in model organisms. Remarkably, rapamycin demonstrated the ability to extend the lifespan of yeast, worms, flies, and mice. These findings ignited interest in the compound as a potential anti-aging agent. The interaction between rapamycin and the mTOR pathway provided insights into the molecular mechanisms of aging and presented a promising target for interventions in the aging process.

Today, rapamycin and its derivatives, often referred to as "rapalogs," are the subject of intensive research in the fields of aging and age-related diseases. While its journey from a remote island's soil to modern laboratories seems serendipitous, it underscores the unpredictable and exciting nature of scientific discovery.

In summary, the discovery of rapamycin is a testament to the serendipity and unpredictability of science. What started as a mere soil sample from a distant island evolved into a story of a compound with transformative potential in medicine and aging research. As we delve deeper into the implications of rapamycin in lifespan extension, it's essential to remember its unique origins and the vast potential that exists in the natural world awaiting discovery.

Significance of Rapamycin in Lifespan Studies

Rapamycin's emergence in the arena of lifespan studies marked a paradigm shift in our understanding of aging and the potential to intervene in the process. The compound's impact on the mTOR pathway, coupled with its observed effects on longevity in multiple organisms, has firmly positioned it as a beacon of promise in the pursuit of extended healthspan and lifespan.

Rapamycin's Universality Across Species

One of the most compelling aspects of rapamycin's significance lies in its universal effects across a variety of organisms. From simple yeast cells to more complex mammals like mice, rapamycin consistently demonstrates an ability to extend lifespan. Such universal efficacy suggests that the mTOR pathway, which rapamycin targets, may play a fundamental and conserved role in aging across diverse species. This universality brings hope that findings in model organisms might translate to benefits in humans.

Shifting the Focus to Healthspan

While the extension of lifespan is a captivating outcome, the broader significance of rapamycin might rest in its potential to enhance healthspan – the period during which an individual remains healthy and free from serious age-related ailments. Studies have indicated that rapamycin not only lengthens life but can also delay the onset of age-related diseases in mice, such as cancer and cognitive decline. Thus, rapamycin offers a two-fold promise: living longer and living healthier.

A Window into the Molecular Mechanisms of Aging

Before the spotlight on rapamycin, the molecular underpinnings of aging were largely enigmatic. The compound's interaction with the mTOR pathway provided researchers with a tangible target to explore the intricacies of cellular aging. By understanding how rapamycin influences mTOR and, in turn, how mTOR affects cellular processes like protein synthesis, growth, and autophagy, scientists have gained valuable insights into the potential drivers of aging. This knowledge can inform future interventions, both pharmacological and perhaps even lifestyle-based, to promote longevity.

A Catalyst for Aging Research

Rapamycin's impact on lifespan studies extends beyond its direct effects. Its discovery galvanized the field, attracting interest from researchers, funding agencies, and biotech companies. The buzz around rapamycin spurred investments in aging research and led to the exploration of other potential lifespan-extending compounds. The compound has, in many ways, served as a catalyst, accelerating progress in a field that seeks to understand one of life's most profound mysteries.

Towards Personalized Longevity Interventions

Rapamycin's significance also extends into the realm of personalized medicine. As researchers delve deeper into its effects, there's growing recognition that individual genetic, metabolic, and other factors might influence responsiveness to the drug. This opens avenues for tailoring anti-aging interventions, ensuring optimal outcomes for individuals based on their unique biological makeup.

In conclusion, the significance of rapamycin in lifespan studies is multifaceted. Beyond its direct, tangible effects on longevity in various organisms, its discovery has reshaped the trajectory of aging research, offering insights into the molecular dance that governs aging, galvanizing the scientific community, and hinting at the tantalizing possibility of personalized longevity interventions. As we navigate the complexities of aging and the potential to extend the boundaries of life, rapamycin stands as a testament to the profound impact that a single compound can have on reshaping our understanding of a fundamental aspect of existence.

Chapter 2:
Background on Rapamycin

Natural Origins and Initial Discovery

The story of rapamycin is deeply intertwined with the rich tapestry of nature and the serendipity of scientific exploration. It underscores the fact that some of the most transformative discoveries often originate from the unlikeliest of sources.

Easter Island: A Place of Mystery and Wonder

Easter Island, or Rapa Nui as it's known locally, is one of the most isolated inhabited islands on Earth, located over 2,000 miles from the nearest population center. Famous for its monumental stone statues, called moai, the island has long been a symbol of mystery and ancient civilization. But beneath the shadow of these stone giants, the soil of Rapa Nui held secrets that would revolutionize modern medicine.

Expedition and Discovery

In 1964, a team of Canadian scientists embarked on a journey to this remote island. Their mission wasn't directly tied to the statues or the island's history. Instead, they were there as part of a broader initiative to collect soil samples from various parts of the world. The goal was to explore the soil's microbial inhabitants, searching for organisms that might produce substances with therapeutic potential.

Amid the collected samples from Rapa Nui, scientists identified a previously unknown bacterium, which they named *Streptomyces hygroscopicus*. This bacterium, as subsequent laboratory tests would reveal, produced a unique compound that demonstrated robust anti-fungal properties. Honoring the island of its origin, the compound was named "rapamycin."

From Antifungal to Immunomodulator

Initially, the scientific community's interest in rapamycin was centered on its potential as an antifungal agent. However, as is often the case in research, unexpected properties emerged. During laboratory tests, rapamycin revealed potent immunosuppressive activities. This meant that it could potentially dampen or modulate the immune response, a property that could be harnessed in various medical scenarios, particularly in preventing the rejection of transplanted organs.

This serendipitous finding shifted the trajectory of rapamycin research. While its antifungal potential took a backseat, its immunomodulatory properties became the focal point of scientific investigations. Rapamycin's journey had taken a fascinating turn, from a soil sample on a remote island to the cusp of medical breakthroughs.

Rapa Nui's Legacy

While rapamycin's discovery is a testament to scientific curiosity and the unpredictability of research, it also highlights the invaluable treasure trove that is our natural world. Nature, with its vast array of organisms, has evolved an incredible array of molecules and compounds, many of which have the potential to benefit humanity in ways yet to be discovered. Rapamycin stands as a shining example of this, a beacon of hope unearthed from the soil of an island better known for ancient stone statues than modern medical marvels.

In essence, the story of rapamycin's natural origins and initial discovery is a powerful reminder of two things: first, that nature remains an unparalleled source of inspiration and solutions for modern challenges, and second, that the path of scientific discovery, much like the moai pathways of Rapa Nui, is often winding, unexpected, but ultimately leads to profound insights that can reshape our understanding of the world and ourselves.

Pharmacological Uses

Rapamycin, once discovered in the soils of Easter Island, quickly transitioned from a compound of interest to a pharmacological marvel. Its multifaceted interactions within the body have led to various therapeutic applications, ranging from immunosuppression to anti-cancer treatments. This chapter delves into the broad spectrum of rapamycin's pharmacological uses and its transformative impact on medicine.

Immunosuppression: A Boon for Organ Transplants

The initial and perhaps most well-known application of rapamycin is its role in immunosuppression. After organ transplantation, the recipient's immune system often recognizes the new organ as foreign, leading to an immune response that can result in organ rejection. Rapamycin, by suppressing certain functions of the immune system, helps prevent this rejection.

Trade names like Sirolimus are commonly prescribed to kidney transplant recipients. Its ability to dampen the immune response without causing nephrotoxicity, a common side effect of many other immunosuppressants, makes it especially valuable in this context.

Anti-Cancer Properties: Targeting Cellular Growth

The mTOR pathway, which rapamycin inhibits, is pivotal in regulating cell growth and proliferation. Some cancers are characterized by dys-regulated mTOR signaling, leading to unchecked cellular growth. By inhibiting mTOR, rapamycin can halt the growth of such cancer cells.

Clinical trials have explored rapamycin and its derivatives (rapalogs) for various cancers, including renal cell carcinoma, breast cancer, and neuroendocrine tumors. The drug's ability to target the metabolic aspects of cancer growth offers a unique therapeutic angle, distinguishing it from traditional chemotherapies.

Anti-Atherosclerosis: Preventing Vascular Diseases

Beyond its role in transplantation and cancer, rapamycin has demonstrated potential in vascular biology. Its anti-proliferative properties can prevent the narrowing of blood vessels, a process that underlies conditions like atherosclerosis. Drug-eluting stents, which are used to keep coronary arteries open after angioplasty, sometimes use rapamycin to prevent restenosis (re-narrowing) of the artery.

Age-Related Diseases: A Glimpse into Potential Applications

Given rapamycin's impact on aging in model organisms, researchers are keen to explore its potential in combatting age-related diseases in humans. Preliminary research suggests that it might play a role in neuroprotective strategies against conditions like Alzheimer's disease. By targeting the mTOR pathway, rapamycin could mitigate some of the detrimental cellular processes associated with aging that contribute to neurological decline.

Safety and Side Effects: A Note of Caution

While rapamycin's pharmacological potential is vast, it's crucial to understand that its suppression of mTOR can lead to side effects. These can range from metabolic disturbances, like elevated blood sugars, to increased susceptibility to infections due to its immunosuppressive nature. Therefore, the therapeutic use of rapamycin requires careful consideration of its risk-benefit profile for each patient.

In conclusion, rapamycin's journey from a soil-derived compound to a pharmacological agent with myriad applications is nothing short of remarkable. Its ability to modulate the immune system, halt cellular growth, and potentially combat age-related diseases positions it as a versatile tool in the medicinal arsenal. As with any drug, its promise is balanced by its risks, but the breadth of rapamycin's pharmacological uses serves as a testament to its profound impact on medicine and its potential to shape therapeutic strategies for a diverse array of conditions.

Molecular Mechanism of Action

Rapamycin's profound impact on diverse biological processes stems from its intricate molecular mechanism of action. Central to this is the mTOR (mechanistic target of rapamycin) pathway, a key regulatory hub in cells. This chapter delves into rapamycin's molecular interactions, demystifying how a single compound can influence such a wide array of physiological outcomes.

mTOR: The Central Player

At the heart of rapamycin's mechanism of action lies mTOR, a serine/threonine protein kinase. mTOR plays a pivotal role in cellular processes, orchestrating responses to various stimuli like nutrients, growth factors, and energy status. It acts as a cellular sensor, integrating these signals to regulate processes like protein synthesis, cell growth, and autophagy.

mTOR exists in two distinct complexes: mTORC1 and mTORC2. While both are important, rapamycin primarily interacts with mTORC1.

Rapamycin's Direct Target: FKBP12

Interestingly, rapamycin doesn't bind directly to mTOR. Instead, it first binds to an intracellular protein called FKBP12 (FK506-binding protein 12). The rapamycin-FKBP12 complex then interacts with mTORC1, inhibiting its activity. This indirect mechanism is crucial, as it ensures specificity and reduces potential off-target effects.

Regulation of Protein Synthesis

One of the primary cellular processes governed by mTORC1 is protein synthesis. By sensing the availability of nutrients and growth factors, mTORC1 can modulate the translation machinery of the cell. When mTORC1 is active, it promotes protein synthesis by phosphorylating key translation initiators, like the S6 kinase and the eIF4E-binding protein.

Rapamycin's inhibition of mTORC1 dampens this protein synthesis machinery, leading to reduced cellular growth and proliferation – a mechanism of particular interest in cancer therapy.

Autophagy: Cellular Recycling

Autophagy, often termed cellular "recycling," is another process regulated by mTORC1. During autophagy, cells degrade damaged proteins and organelles, using the recycled components as building blocks. This process is essential for cellular health and homeostasis.

mTORC1 typically inhibits autophagy under nutrient-rich conditions. However, when rapamycin inhibits mTORC1, autophagy is promoted. This has implications for aging and neurodegenerative diseases, where enhanced autophagy can be beneficial.

Cell Growth and Metabolism

Beyond protein synthesis and autophagy, mTORC1 also regulates cell growth by modulating lipid synthesis and glycolysis. Rapamycin, through mTORC1 inhibition, can alter the metabolic profile of cells, which is of interest in conditions like cancer, where metabolic reprogramming is a hallmark.

Implications of mTORC2 Interactions

While rapamycin's primary target is mTORC1, prolonged exposure can also impact mTORC2, although this interaction is less understood. mTORC2 plays roles in cell survival, metabolism, and the cytoskeleton. The implications of rapamycin's potential effects on mTORC2 are areas of ongoing research.

In summary, the molecular dance between rapamycin, FKBP12, and the mTOR complexes underscores the compound's vast physiological reach. Its ability to modulate the mTOR pathway, a central integrator of cellular signals, positions rapamycin as a potent regulator of cell growth, metabolism, and survival. This molecular mechanism of action provides a foundation for understanding rapamycin's diverse therapeutic applications and its promising role in conditions ranging from cancer to age-related diseases. As researchers continue to dissect these interactions, we gain deeper insights into cellular regulation and the potential to harness these pathways for therapeutic benefit.

Chapter 3:
Rapamycin and Aging:
The Research Journey

Early Observations in Yeast and Simple Organisms

The journey of understanding rapamycin's influence on lifespan and cellular health began, intriguingly, in the world of microscopic organisms. From the single-celled budding yeast to more complex organisms like nematodes and fruit flies, these early observations laid the groundwork for the more advanced studies that would follow. Let's explore how rapamycin first hinted at its potential through these simple life forms.

Yeast: The Model Microorganism

Budding yeast, or *Saccharomyces cerevisiae*, has been a cornerstone of biological research due to its simplicity and the conservation of many of its cellular pathways with higher organisms. The TOR (Target Of Rapamycin) pathway, for which mTOR in mammals is named, was first characterized in yeast.

When scientists exposed yeast cells to rapamycin, they noticed a significant extension in lifespan. More intriguingly, these yeast cells also displayed a delay in age-related cellular decline, suggesting that not only was rapamycin influencing lifespan, but it was also promoting "healthspan."

Nematodes: The Tiny Worm with Big Answers

C. elegans, a transparent nematode, is another favorite model organism in aging research. When researchers administered rapamycin to these worms, a consistent extension of lifespan was observed. Moreover, the treated nematodes retained their mobility and physiological health for a more significant portion of their lives.

This observation in a multicellular organism reinforced the idea that the effects of rapamycin might not be limited to single-celled life forms but could translate to more complex beings.

Fruit Flies: From Yeast to Flight

Drosophila melanogaster, commonly known as the fruit fly, was next in line to reveal rapamycin's secrets. Once again, the results were consistent. Fruit flies exposed to rapamycin exhibited an extended lifespan. But beyond just living longer, these flies showed signs of improved health. They retained their mobility and reproductive capabilities for a more extended period, suggesting that rapamycin was not only extending life but enhancing its quality.

Unraveling the Mechanisms

With consistent observations across diverse organisms, scientists were eager to unravel the underpinnings. A common thread emerged: the inhibition of the TOR pathway, which, as in mammals, played a crucial role in regulating growth and metabolism in these simpler organisms.

In yeast, the downregulation of the TOR pathway led to a state akin to caloric restriction, a condition known to extend lifespan across multiple species. Similarly, in both nematodes and fruit flies, the suppression of the TOR pathway led to a host of beneficial metabolic changes and stress responses that contributed to their extended vitality.

Implications of Early Findings

The consistent lifespan-extending effects of rapamycin across such a wide phylogenetic range, from yeast to fruit flies, strongly hinted at a fundamental, conserved mechanism at play. These findings fueled optimism that the effects might be replicable in more complex organisms, possibly even mammals.

In summary, while these organisms are far removed from humans in complexity, they share many of the fundamental pathways that govern growth, metabolism, and aging. The early observations of rapamycin's effects in these simple organisms provided the initial glimmers of understanding, hinting at the compound's profound potential. As we delve deeper into rapamycin's journey, these humble beginnings serve as a poignant reminder of how even the simplest life forms can offer insights with vast implications for human health and longevity.

Mammalian Studies

After initial observations in simpler organisms, researchers were eager to explore rapamycin's potential in mammals. These studies would bridge the gap between basic research and potential therapeutic applications for humans. The findings from mammalian studies, particularly in rodents, have been both exciting and illuminating, shedding light on rapamycin's profound influence on mammalian physiology and healthspan.

Mouse Models: Extending Lifespan

Mice, due to their physiological similarities to humans, serve as a primary model for studying human diseases and potential treatments. Initial studies administering rapamycin to mice resulted in a notable finding: a consistent extension of lifespan, even when the treatment started late in life.

Both male and female mice benefited from rapamycin treatment, although the magnitude of lifespan extension varied. This result was groundbreaking. It provided strong evidence that the lifespan-extending effects observed in yeast, worms, and flies could translate to mammals.

Healthspan: Beyond Just Living Longer

Equally important to the extended lifespan was the observation that mice on rapamycin exhibited signs of improved healthspan. These mice showed delayed onset of age-related diseases, maintained lean body mass, and displayed enhanced cognitive function and motor coordination as they aged.

Such observations suggest that rapamycin's impact isn't merely about adding years to life but, more crucially, adding life to those years.

Cardiac Health and Rapamycin

Heart diseases are a primary concern in aging populations. In mice, rapamycin demonstrated a potential protective effect against age-related cardiac diseases. Treated mice showed better heart function and a reduced incidence of age-associated cardiac pathologies.

Cancer Prevention and Rapamycin

Given rapamycin's mechanism of action through mTOR inhibition, researchers hypothesized it might offer protective effects against cancer, as mTOR is often dysregulated in various tumors. Indeed, mice treated with rapamycin exhibited a decreased incidence of cancer and a delay in cancer onset, emphasizing the compound's potential as an anti-cancer agent.

Neuroprotective Effects

Neurodegenerative diseases, such as Alzheimer's, represent another significant concern in aging populations. Preliminary studies in mice suggested that rapamycin could alleviate some symptoms of neurodegenerative diseases and enhance cognitive function.

Potential Downsides: Not All Rosy

While the benefits of rapamycin were evident in multiple studies, researchers also observed potential downsides. Some mice exhibited glucose intolerance, and there were concerns about immunosuppression, given rapamycin's original use as an immunosuppressive drug. These observations emphasized the need for a balanced understanding of rapamycin's effects and potential trade-offs.

Broader Implications for Mammalian Aging

The mammalian studies reinforced a central idea that began in simpler organisms: the mTOR pathway is a conserved regulator of aging. By modulating this pathway, it seems possible to influence the rate of aging and the onset of age-related diseases, at least in controlled settings.

In summary, mammalian studies have been pivotal in advancing our understanding of rapamycin's potential. They offer a glimpse into a future where we might harness the power of molecules like rapamycin to improve healthspan and combat age-related diseases. While the journey from mice to humans is fraught with challenges, these studies lay a robust foundation, fueling hope and curiosity for what lies ahead in the realm of aging and longevity research.

The Challenge of Dosing and Administration in Humans

While the promise of rapamycin in extending lifespan and improving healthspan in simpler organisms and mammals is evident, its translation to human use is not straightforward. One of the primary challenges lies in determining the appropriate dosing and administration for humans. This section delves into these complexities, highlighting the balance between therapeutic benefit and potential side effects.

From Mice to Men: Scaling the Dose

Administering drugs in mice and then extrapolating the dosage to humans is not as simple as adjusting for body weight. Differences in metabolism, drug absorption, distribution, excretion, and other pharmacokinetic factors come into play. For rapamycin, which has a profound impact on fundamental cellular processes, getting the dose right is crucial.

Potential Side Effects at Higher Doses

Rapamycin, initially developed as an immunosuppressant, can lead to reduced immune function at higher doses. In an aging population, where immune function is already compromised, this presents a challenge. There's a fine line between harnessing rapamycin's therapeutic benefits and inadvertently suppressing the immune system to a point of vulnerability.

Moreover, studies have shown that at certain doses, rapamycin might induce glucose intolerance and increase the risk of developing diabetes-like symptoms. These potential side effects underscore the importance of precise dosing.

Finding the Therapeutic Window

The goal in drug administration is always to find the "therapeutic window" – the dose range within which a drug exerts its beneficial effects without causing unacceptable side effects. For rapamycin, this window needs to be defined clearly. Ongoing clinical trials aim to pinpoint this range, but it's a delicate balance, especially considering the long-term administration required for lifespan extension.

Interindividual Variability

Humans exhibit significant variability in their response to drugs. Factors such as genetics, age, diet, and concurrent medications can all influence how an individual responds to a given dose of rapamycin. This variability means that a dose beneficial for one person might be suboptimal or even harmful for another. Personalized dosing, based on individual characteristics and perhaps even genetic makeup, might be the way forward.

Formulation and Delivery

Beyond the actual dose, the formulation of rapamycin and its mode of delivery can influence its effectiveness and side effect profile. Should it be administered orally, intravenously, or in some other form? How frequently should it be given? These are questions researchers grapple with, and the answers could significantly influence rapamycin's therapeutic potential.

Long-term Administration: Uncharted Waters

Considering rapamycin for lifespan extension introduces another challenge: the potential need for long-term or even lifelong administration. The long-term effects of continuous rapamycin administration in humans remain unknown. There's a vast difference between short-term drug treatments for specific diseases and lifelong administration for healthspan enhancement. The safety profile over extended periods remains a crucial area of investigation.

In Conclusion

The therapeutic potential of rapamycin in lifespan extension is undeniably exciting. However, the road to its widespread use in humans is paved with challenges, especially concerning dosing and administration. While the journey is complex, it's one that researchers are ardently pursuing, with the hope that the lessons from simpler organisms and mammals can indeed be translated to enhance human health and longevity. As research progresses, a clearer picture of rapamycin's place in human health will emerge, balancing its profound promise with the practicalities of real-world application.

Chapter 4:
Potential Mechanisms: How Does Rapamycin Influence Aging?

Caloric Restriction Mimicry

Caloric restriction (CR) has long been identified as one of the most consistent interventions to extend lifespan across various organisms, from yeast to primates. It involves reducing daily calorie intake without malnutrition, resulting in a host of metabolic and physiological changes that confer health and longevity benefits. Rapamycin, with its profound effects on cellular pathways, has been explored as a potential "caloric restriction mimetic" (CRM). This chapter dives into the concept of caloric restriction mimicry and how rapamycin might simulate some of CR's beneficial effects without the need for dietary restriction.

The Magic of Caloric Restriction

CR's ability to extend lifespan is remarkable. In organisms subjected to CR, there's not just an extension of life but a delay in the onset of age-related diseases, improved stress resistance, and enhanced metabolic health. But what underlies these benefits?

On a cellular level, CR leads to reduced oxidative stress, enhanced autophagy (cellular "clean-up" processes), and changes in energy metabolism. These changes collectively contribute to improved cellular function and resistance to age-related decline.

The Challenge of Dietary Restriction in Humans

While CR's benefits are well-documented, its practical application in humans is challenging. Long-term caloric restriction requires significant dietary discipline and may not be feasible or desirable for many. Additionally, potential downsides, such as reduced muscle mass or bone density, and the impact on reproductive health, present concerns.

Hence, the search for compounds that can mimic the benefits of CR without the need for reduced food intake is of immense interest. Enter rapamycin.

Rapamycin: A Caloric Restriction Mimetic?

Rapamycin's effects on the mTOR pathway have parallels with some of the cellular changes observed during CR. By inhibiting mTOR, rapamycin can replicate several metabolic and stress response adaptations seen in organisms on a restricted diet.

For instance, both CR and rapamycin treatment enhance autophagy, the process by which cells break down and recycle damaged components. Enhanced autophagy is believed to play a crucial role in maintaining cellular health and preventing age-related decline.

Similarly, both interventions lead to a shift in cellular metabolism, favoring lipid oxidation and increased mitochondrial efficiency. This metabolic shift is thought to reduce oxidative stress, a significant contributor to cellular aging.

Differences Between CR and Rapamycin Treatment

While there are similarities, it's essential to recognize that rapamycin does not replicate all of CR's effects. For example, while CR typically improves insulin sensitivity, rapamycin, at certain doses, has been shown to impair glucose tolerance. Such differences underscore the need for a nuanced understanding of rapamycin's role as a CRM.

The Promise of CR Mimicry

The allure of CR mimicry lies in the potential to harness the health and longevity benefits of caloric restriction without the challenges of dietary adherence. If compounds like rapamycin can effectively mimic a significant fraction of CR's benefits, it opens the door to a novel approach to healthspan enhancement.

In Conclusion

Caloric restriction's profound impact on lifespan and healthspan has driven the search for interventions that can replicate its benefits without the associated dietary challenges. Rapamycin, with its effects on pathways that overlap with those modulated by CR, emerges as a promising candidate for caloric restriction mimicry. While not a perfect match, its potential to enhance health and longevity, echoing some of CR's magic, makes it a compelling focus of longevity research. As we continue to understand rapamycin's role in this context, the dream of harnessing the benefits of dietary restriction without the sacrifice comes ever closer to reality.

Reduction of Cellular Senescence

Cellular senescence, the state where cells lose their ability to divide and function efficiently, plays a critical role in the aging process and the onset of age-related diseases. These senescent cells, while no longer proliferative, remain metabolically active and often secrete inflammatory molecules that can negatively influence their neighboring cells. In the quest for longevity and improved healthspan, reducing or managing cellular senescence emerges as a pivotal strategy. This chapter explores the relationship between rapamycin and the reduction of cellular senescence.

The Phenomenon of Cellular Senescence

Originally identified as a barrier to unlimited cell division in culture, cellular senescence was later recognized as a potent tumor-suppressive mechanism. While stopping rogue cells from proliferating uncontrollably is beneficial, there's a trade-off. Over time, the accumulation of senescent cells in tissues can lead to chronic inflammation, tissue dysfunction, and a host of age-related diseases.

The 'SASP' Factor

One of the defining features of senescent cells is the Senescence-Associated Secretory Phenotype (SASP). This involves the secretion of pro-inflammatory cytokines, growth factors, and proteases. While SASP can have beneficial roles in wound healing and tissue repair, chronic SASP contributes to tissue damage and can promote tumorigenesis.

Rapamycin and Cellular Senescence

Given rapamycin's broad effects on cellular metabolism and growth, its impact on cellular senescence is of great interest. Here's how rapamycin interfaces with the senescence landscape:

1. **Inhibition of mTOR and Senescence Prevention:** By inhibiting the mTOR pathway, rapamycin can delay the onset of cellular senescence. This delay means fewer senescent cells in tissues, translating to reduced inflammation and improved tissue function.

2. **Reduction of the SASP:** Some studies suggest that rapamycin can attenuate the SASP. By reducing the secretion of pro-inflammatory molecules from senescent cells, rapamycin might mitigate the negative paracrine effects of these cells on their environment.

3. **Promotion of Autophagy:** Rapamycin's ability to enhance autophagy, the cellular cleanup process, might contribute to the removal of senescent cells. Efficient autophagy can help maintain cellular health and delay the onset of senescence.

Comparing Rapamycin to Senolytics

While rapamycin modulates cellular senescence, it's essential to differentiate its effects from those of senolytics—compounds specifically designed to target and remove senescent cells. Rapamycin primarily delays the onset of senescence and reduces the SASP, while senolytics aim to purge existing senescent cells from tissues. Both approaches have merits and can be complementary in strategies aiming for longevity and healthspan extension.

Challenges and Considerations

While the potential of rapamycin in managing cellular senescence is evident, challenges persist:

- **Optimal Dosing:** As with other effects of rapamycin, determining the optimal dose for reducing cellular senescence without triggering adverse effects remains critical.

- **Long-term Impact:** The long-term effects of continuous mTOR inhibition on cellular health and function need further exploration.

In Conclusion

The reduction of cellular senescence emerges as a promising avenue to combat aging and improve healthspan. Rapamycin, with its profound effects on cellular pathways intertwined with the senescence process, offers a potential tool in this endeavor. While not a silver bullet, its role in modulating cellular senescence further cements its place in the pantheon of potential anti-aging compounds. As research continues, the nuances of rapamycin's interaction with cellular senescence will become clearer, guiding its therapeutic applications in the quest for longevity.

Enhancing Stem Cell Function

Stem cells, with their ability to self-renew and differentiate into various cell types, are cornerstones of tissue repair, regeneration, and overall vitality. As we age, stem cell function declines, leading to diminished tissue repair capacity and the onset of degenerative conditions. There's growing interest in the potential of interventions like rapamycin to enhance stem cell function, thereby bolstering the body's regenerative capabilities and counteracting some of the detrimental effects of aging. This chapter delves into the intricate relationship between rapamycin and stem cell function.

The Role of Stem Cells in Health and Aging

Stem cells are unique in their dual ability: they can both replicate to produce more stem cells and differentiate into specialized cells as needed. Throughout life, they replace damaged or old cells, ensuring tissue maintenance and repair.

However, as we age, stem cell numbers and function decline. This decline is implicated in slower healing rates, reduced organ function, and the onset of various age-associated diseases. Thus, rejuvenating stem cell function could be a key to extending healthspan.

Rapamycin and Stem Cell Rejuvenation

Rapamycin, given its role in regulating cell growth and proliferation through the mTOR pathway, has implications for stem cell biology.

Here's how rapamycin might influence stem cells:

1. **Maintenance of Stem Cell Quiescence:** Stem cells exist in a state of "quiescence" (a dormant state) until activated for repair or turnover. Rapamycin can promote this quiescence, preserving the stem cell pool and preventing premature exhaustion.

2. **Enhancement of Autophagy:** Rapamycin's promotion of autophagy can help in clearing damaged cellular components. For stem cells, this means a cleaner, more efficient cellular environment, potentially enhancing their function and longevity.

3. **Mitigating Age-related Dysfunction:** By inhibiting the mTOR pathway, rapamycin can reverse some of the age-related dysfunctions observed in stem cells, making them more responsive to tissue repair signals.

Empirical Evidence: Studies in Mice

Several studies in mice have demonstrated the potential of rapamycin in enhancing stem cell function:

- **Hematopoietic Stem Cells (HSCs):** These are the stem cells responsible for the generation of all blood cell types. Rapamycin treatment has been shown to rejuvenate aged HSCs, enhancing their function and improving blood formation.
- **Muscle Stem Cells:** In the context of skeletal muscle regeneration, rapamycin can improve the function of aged muscle stem cells, aiding in better muscle repair.

Potential Applications in Regenerative Medicine

The ability of rapamycin to rejuvenate stem cell function has profound implications for regenerative medicine. It could be used as a pre-treatment for stem cell therapies, ensuring the cells are in their optimal state before transplantation. Moreover, in conditions where tissue regeneration is essential, like after injuries or surgeries, rapamycin could potentially expedite the healing process.

Challenges and Caveats

While the potential is vast, there are challenges:

- **Dosing and Timing:** The optimal dose and timing of rapamycin administration for stem cell rejuvenation need to be delineated.
- **Unintended Consequences:** Continuous mTOR inhibition might have unintended consequences, including possible effects on stem cell differentiation.

In Conclusion

Stem cells stand at the forefront of our body's regenerative capabilities. Enhancing their function, especially as we age, could dramatically improve health outcomes and longevity. Rapamycin, with its multifaceted interaction with cellular pathways crucial for stem cell function, emerges as a promising agent in this realm. As research deepens, we might find ourselves on the cusp of harnessing rapamycin's full potential in stem cell biology, revolutionizing our approach to healthspan extension and regenerative medicine.

Modulation of Inflammation and Immunity

Inflammation and immunity are two tightly intertwined systems. While inflammation is a protective response to injury or infection, chronic inflammation is a hallmark of aging, known as "inflammaging," and can drive numerous age-related diseases. Immunity, on the other hand, protects the body from foreign invaders. However, as we age, immune responses can become dysregulated, leading to increased susceptibility to infections and diseases. Rapamycin, with its broad effects on cellular metabolism and growth, has intriguing implications for both inflammation and immunity. This chapter explores rapamycin's role in modulating these crucial physiological processes.

The Double-edged Sword of Inflammation

Inflammation is essentially the body's response to stressors, be they physical injuries, infections, or harmful agents. It involves the activation of immune cells, the release of signaling molecules (cytokines), and tissue repair mechanisms. However, when inflammation becomes chronic or systemic, it's more harmful than protective, contributing to various conditions from cardiovascular diseases to neurodegenerative disorders.

Rapamycin's Anti-inflammatory Effects

Rapamycin has demonstrated potent anti-inflammatory effects, which can be attributed to several mechanisms:

1. **mTOR Inhibition:** mTOR signaling is associated with the production of various inflammatory cytokines. By inhibiting mTOR, rapamycin can dampen inflammatory responses.

2. **Reduction of the SASP:** As previously discussed, senescent cells often secrete pro-inflammatory compounds, known as the Senescence-Associated Secretory Phenotype (SASP). Rapamycin can mitigate this secretion, reducing inflammation at the cellular level.

3. **Promotion of Autophagy:** Enhanced autophagy, stimulated by rapamycin, can lead to the clearance of damaged cellular components that might otherwise trigger inflammatory responses.

Rapamycin and Immune Modulation

Aging is associated with immune system decline, termed "immunosenescence." This decline manifests as reduced vaccine responses, increased susceptibility to infections, and a higher risk of autoimmune disorders. Rapamycin's interaction with the immune system is multifaceted:

1. **Enhancement of Immune Memory:** Studies have shown that rapamycin can improve the function of memory T cells, which are pivotal for long-lasting immunity against previously encountered pathogens.

2. **Rejuvenation of Immune Repertoire:** Rapamycin can rejuvenate the diversity of immune cells, especially in the aged environment, potentially restoring a more youthful immune response.

3. **Balancing Immune Responses:** By modulating mTOR signaling, rapamycin can promote a balance between different immune cell types, ensuring that responses are neither too weak (leading to infections) nor too strong (causing autoimmunity).

Clinical Implications

Given rapamycin's effects on inflammation and immunity, there are exciting clinical implications:

- **Age-related Diseases:** Rapamycin's anti-inflammatory properties can be harnessed in treating or preventing diseases driven by chronic inflammation.
- **Vaccination in the Elderly:** Enhancing immune responses using rapamycin might improve vaccine efficacy in older individuals.
- **Autoimmune Disorders:** By balancing immune responses, rapamycin could be explored as a treatment for autoimmune conditions.

Challenges and Future Directions

While the potential benefits of rapamycin in modulating inflammation and immunity are evident, challenges remain:

- **Optimal Dosing:** Determining the right dose for immune modulation without compromising the body's defense mechanisms is crucial.
- **Long-term Effects:** Continuous modulation of immune responses might have unforeseen consequences that need thorough investigation.

In Conclusion

Inflammation and immunity, integral to health and aging, stand as promising targets for interventions like rapamycin. By understanding and harnessing rapamycin's modulatory effects on these systems, we might be better equipped to combat age-related decline and diseases, inching closer to the goal of extended healthspan and quality of life.

Chapter 5:
Challenges and Controversies

Potential Side Effects and Drawbacks

While the prospects of rapamycin in lifespan extension and health improvement are tantalizing, no intervention is without its caveats. Rapamycin, though promising, comes with its array of potential side effects and drawbacks. A comprehensive understanding of these is imperative for making informed decisions about its use and for future research endeavors. This chapter elucidates the potential downsides and challenges associated with rapamycin administration.

Rapamycin's Origins in Immunosuppression

It's pivotal to remember that rapamycin was initially developed as an immunosuppressant, primarily used to prevent organ transplant rejection. This very property implies that there are inherent risks in its long-term or widespread use:

1. **Increased Infection Risk:** By dampening immune responses, rapamycin can potentially increase susceptibility to infections. This is especially concerning for the elderly or those with compromised immune systems.

2. **Potential for Autoimmunity:** Paradoxically, while rapamycin suppresses certain immune functions, it might enhance others, potentially leading to autoimmune reactions.

Metabolic Concerns

Rapamycin's interaction with the mTOR pathway, which plays a key role in metabolism, can lead to several metabolic concerns:

1. **Insulin Resistance:** Some studies have suggested that rapamycin might induce insulin resistance, a precursor to type 2 diabetes.

2. **Lipid Profile Alteration:** Changes in cholesterol and triglyceride levels have been noted in some individuals taking rapamycin.

Wound Healing and Regeneration

Given its origins as an anti-proliferative agent, rapamycin could potentially interfere with processes that require rapid cell division:

1. **Delayed Wound Healing:** Rapamycin might slow down the wound healing process, which relies on swift cell proliferation and migration.

2. **Potential Impact on Pregnancy:** The implications of rapamycin on fetal development and pregnancy are not entirely clear, but caution is advised given the drug's potential anti-proliferative effects.

Neurological and Cognitive Effects

While research is still in its infancy, some potential neurological concerns associated with rapamycin include:

1. **Mood Alterations:** Some animal studies have shown that rapamycin might influence behaviors linked to anxiety and depression.

2. **Potential Cognitive Impact:** While some studies suggest rapamycin might be protective against neurodegenerative diseases, its long-term impact on cognitive function requires further exploration.

Chronic Inhibition Concerns

Continuous mTOR inhibition might have unforeseen consequences:

1. **Loss of mTOR's Beneficial Roles:** While mTOR is associated with aging and disease, it also has essential roles in growth, memory, and learning. Chronic inhibition might inadvertently suppress these beneficial effects.

2. **Unexplored Long-term Effects:** The consequences of lifelong mTOR pathway suppression in humans remain largely uncharted territory.

Formulation and Delivery Challenges

The delivery of rapamycin presents its own set of challenges:

1. **Bioavailability:** The oral bioavailability of rapamycin can vary, potentially leading to inconsistent effects.

2. **Interactions with Other Drugs:** As with any medication, there's potential for adverse interactions when rapamycin is taken with other drugs.

In Conclusion

The allure of rapamycin as a potential anti-aging intervention is undeniable. However, like any powerful tool, it comes with risks and drawbacks that need careful consideration. Balancing the potential benefits against these challenges is the key to harnessing rapamycin's power safely and effectively. As we move forward, meticulous research and clinical trials will be instrumental in delineating rapamycin's true potential and pitfalls in the realm of health and longevity.

Ethics of Lifespan Extension

The quest for the proverbial fountain of youth, or in modern terms, interventions like rapamycin that promise lifespan extension, inevitably stirs profound ethical debates. While the idea of living longer, healthier lives is undoubtedly appealing, it raises numerous questions about the nature of human existence, societal implications, and the very definition of life itself. This chapter seeks to untangle some of the intricate ethical threads woven into the fabric of lifespan extension.

The Right to Longevity

At the core of the debate lies a fundamental question: Do humans have a right to extended life?

1. **Personal Autonomy:** Some argue that individuals have the right to make decisions about their bodies, which includes the choice to use interventions that extend life. It's an extension of the personal freedom to make health decisions.

2. **Natural Order of Things:** Conversely, others believe that there's a natural lifespan for organisms, including humans, and that artificially extending it might be playing with the very essence of existence.

Societal Implications

Lifespan extension, if widely available, could have profound effects on society:

1. **Overpopulation:** One of the chief concerns is the potential strain on resources due to overpopulation. If a significant proportion of the population lives much longer, it could lead to challenges related to housing, food, and environmental sustainability.

2. **Economic Impact:** Longer lives could mean prolonged careers, which might have implications for job markets, retirement ages, and pension systems.

3. **Social Dynamics:** Multi-generational living might become the norm, impacting family structures, inheritance customs, and generational dynamics.

Distribution and Access

Any discussion about a medical intervention invariably touches on issues of access and distribution:

1. **Equity:** If lifespan-extending interventions become available, who gets access? Is it only the wealthy, thereby widening the gap between the rich and the poor? Or can it be universally accessible, ensuring everyone benefits?

2. **Medical Prioritization:** Should resources be channeled towards lifespan extension when there are still numerous diseases without cures? How do we prioritize medical research and funding?

Quality vs. Quantity of Life

It's crucial to differentiate between merely extending life and enhancing its quality:

1. **Morbidity:** What if the extended life comes with prolonged periods of illness or diminished capacity? The focus should ideally be on healthspan (disease-free life) rather than just lifespan.

2. **Mental Health Implications:** Living longer might have unforeseen psychological implications. The mental toll of seeing multiple generations pass, the potential loneliness or existential crises need consideration.

Playing God

A deeply philosophical aspect of the debate revolves around the concept of "playing God":

1. **Ethical Boundaries in Science:** Just because we can, does it mean we should? Where do we draw the line in manipulating the natural processes of life and death?

2. **Religious Implications:** Many religious beliefs have defined views on life, death, and the afterlife. Lifespan extension might challenge or conflict with these beliefs.

In Conclusion

The potential of rapamycin and other lifespan-extending interventions takes us into uncharted ethical waters. While the science advances, society must grapple with the philosophical, moral, and practical implications of extended life. A collective, inclusive discourse is essential, ensuring that the path to longevity remains ethically sound, equitable, and truly beneficial to humanity.

Differences in Efficacy Among Populations

As with many medical interventions, the efficacy of rapamycin in extending lifespan and improving health might vary among diverse populations. Factors such as genetics, environmental influences, diet, and pre-existing health conditions can all play a role in how individuals respond to treatments. Understanding these differences is crucial for tailoring interventions, ensuring safety, and maximizing benefits. This chapter delves into the variability of rapamycin's efficacy among different groups.

Genetic Factors

1. **Genetic Variability:** Human populations have diverse genetic backgrounds that can influence drug metabolism, efficacy, and potential side effects. Genetic polymorphisms in the mTOR pathway or related processes could modulate rapamycin's effects.

2. **Ancestral Lineages:** Certain ancestral lineages might carry genetic factors that either potentiate or diminish the benefits of rapamycin. Research on genetically diverse cohorts is essential to understand these nuances.

Dietary and Environmental Influences

1. **Dietary Interactions:** The efficacy of rapamycin might be influenced by dietary habits. For instance, diets rich in certain nutrients might either complement or counteract rapamycin's actions.

2. **Environmental Stressors:** Chronic exposure to environmental stressors, such as pollutants or radiation, could modify the effects of rapamycin on lifespan and health.

Age and Life Stage

1. **Pediatric vs. Adult vs. Elderly:** Rapamycin's impact might differ based on life stages. For instance, its effects in children, who are still growing and developing, might be distinct from its effects in adults or the elderly.

2. **Hormonal Influences:** Life stages marked by hormonal changes, like puberty or menopause, might interact with rapamycin's mechanisms, altering its efficacy.

Sex Differences

1. **Physiological Variations:** Men and women have inherent physiological differences that can influence drug metabolism and effects. Hormonal profiles, fat distribution, and organ function variability can all play a role.

2. **Sex-specific Health Concerns:** Some conditions are more prevalent in one sex over the other. For instance, the risk of osteoporosis in postmenopausal women might interact with rapamycin's effects on bone health.

Pre-existing Health Conditions

1. **Metabolic Conditions:** Individuals with metabolic disorders, such as diabetes or obesity, might experience different outcomes with rapamycin due to altered metabolic pathways.

2. **Immune Status:** As an immunomodulator, rapamycin's effects could be distinct in individuals with immune disorders, either autoimmune in nature or immunodeficiency states.

Socioeconomic and Cultural Differences

1. **Access to Healthcare:** Socioeconomic factors can influence access to regular medical care, which might modulate the long-term efficacy of rapamycin. Regular monitoring and dose adjustments, if needed, play a crucial role in treatment outcomes.

2. **Cultural Beliefs:** Some cultures might have beliefs or practices that influence the use of medicines or adherence to treatment. Cultural understanding is pivotal to ensure optimal outcomes.

In Conclusion

While the promise of rapamycin in lifespan extension is universal, its application and outcomes might be nuanced based on diverse population factors. Recognizing these differences is not only vital for personalized medicine but also for ensuring equitable access and benefits for all. Future research endeavors should prioritize diverse cohorts, ensuring that the science of longevity is as inclusive and comprehensive as possible.

Economic Implications of a Longer-Living Population

The idea of a population living significantly longer lives, made possible by interventions like rapamycin, has profound economic implications. Such a demographic shift would reverberate through every facet of the economy, from the workforce and pensions to healthcare and housing. This chapter seeks to unpack some of the multifaceted economic ramifications of a longer-living population.

Labor Market and Employment

1. **Extended Working Lives:** A longer lifespan could equate to an extended working life. This might lead to a delay in retirement, with individuals choosing to or needing to remain in the workforce longer.

2. **Generational Job Competition:** With more generations active in the labor market simultaneously, there could be increased competition for jobs, especially entry-level positions. This might pose challenges for younger individuals entering the job market.

3. **Skill Evolution and Training:** Prolonged careers might necessitate continuous skill evolution. The demand for lifelong learning and periodic retraining might surge.

Pension Systems and Retirement Funds

1. **Solvency Concerns:** Pension systems, both public and private, are predicated on actuarial assumptions of life expectancy. A sudden surge in lifespan could strain these systems, threatening their solvency.

2. **Adjustment of Retirement Age:** To counteract the strain on pension systems, retirement ages might need upward revision.

3. **Personal Savings:** Individuals might need to rethink personal retirement savings strategies, given the possibility of living longer post-retirement.

Healthcare Costs and Infrastructure

1. **Shift in Healthcare Needs:** While lifespan might increase, it's essential to discern whether this equates to a longer healthspan. If not, there could be a significant increase in the geriatric population with chronic illnesses, demanding prolonged healthcare support.

2. **Medical Infrastructure:** The healthcare infrastructure might need expansion or reorientation to cater to the needs of an older population, from specialized facilities to geriatric care professionals.

3. **Insurance Implications:** Health and life insurance paradigms would need recalibration. Premium structures, coverage plans, and policy terms might all undergo transformations.

Real Estate and Housing

1. **Multi-Generational Housing:** With extended family structures, there might be a shift towards multi-generational housing. Real estate designs might evolve to accommodate such living arrangements.

2. **Senior Living Facilities:** The demand for senior living communities or assisted living facilities could grow, necessitating more investment in this sector.

Education and Skill Development

1. **Lifelong Learning:** With extended lives and careers, the education system might transition towards a model that supports continuous learning, accommodating periodic skill upgrades.

2. **Diverse Age Groups:** Educational institutions might witness a more diverse age group of learners, from young adults to seniors.

Consumption Patterns

1. **Evolving Demands:** A longer-living population might have different consumption preferences, impacting industries ranging from travel and leisure to consumer goods.

2. **Economic Growth:** Increased longevity could lead to sustained economic activity and potentially boost growth, given the extended consumer and workforce participation.

In Conclusion

The economic landscape in a world with extended human lifespans would be markedly different from what we know today. While the prospect carries a host of challenges, it also presents opportunities for innovation, growth, and societal evolution. Forward-looking policies, adaptive business strategies, and inclusive societal frameworks will be key in navigating this brave new world of longevity.

Chapter 6: Broader Impacts of Rapamycin on Health

Effects on Neurodegeneration

Neurodegenerative diseases, including Alzheimer's, Parkinson's, and Huntington's, are characterized by the progressive loss of structure or function of neurons. One of the most tantalizing prospects in the study of rapamycin and its derivatives is their potential effect on neurodegeneration. This chapter delves into what we currently understand about rapamycin's impact on neurodegenerative processes and disorders.

Molecular Mechanisms

1. **Autophagy Activation:** One of rapamycin's primary actions is the stimulation of autophagy, a cellular "clean-up" mechanism. In the context of the nervous system, enhanced autophagy can help in the removal of aberrant proteins, often implicated in neurodegenerative diseases.

2. **mTOR Pathway Modulation:** By inhibiting the mTOR pathway, rapamycin might influence various cellular processes critical for neuron function and survival.

Alzheimer's Disease

1. **Amyloid-beta Plaque Clearance:** Enhanced autophagy could aid in clearing amyloid-beta plaques, a hallmark of Alzheimer's. Some studies suggest rapamycin's potential in reducing plaque accumulation in the brain.

2. **Neuroinflammation Reduction:** Chronic inflammation is a significant component of Alzheimer's pathology. Rapamycin's anti-inflammatory effects might provide neuroprotective benefits.

Parkinson's Disease

1. **Clearance of Alpha-Synuclein:** Parkinson's is characterized by the accumulation of alpha-synuclein proteins. Rapamycin-mediated autophagy might assist in clearing these protein aggregates, potentially slowing disease progression.

2. **Dopaminergic Neuron Protection:** Preliminary studies suggest that rapamycin might exert protective effects on dopaminergic neurons, the primary neuronal type affected in Parkinson's.

Huntington's Disease

1. **Huntingtin Protein Aggregate Removal:** Huntington's disease arises from a mutant huntingtin protein. Enhancing autophagy via rapamycin could help remove these toxic proteins, offering therapeutic benefits.

2. **Neurotrophic Support:** There's evidence suggesting rapamycin might enhance the production or action of neurotrophic factors, essential for neuron health, which could be beneficial in conditions like Huntington's.

General Neuroprotective Effects

1. **Oxidative Stress Mitigation:** Rapamycin might provide protection against oxidative stress, a key contributor to neuronal damage in various neurodegenerative conditions.

2. **Brain-Derived Neurotrophic Factor (BDNF) Enhancement:** BDNF plays a crucial role in neuronal survival, growth, and differentiation. Some evidence suggests rapamycin might elevate BDNF levels, providing neuroprotection.

Challenges and Considerations

1. **Brain Bioavailability:** For rapamycin to be effective in treating neurodegenerative conditions, it needs to cross the blood-brain barrier. Current formulations might need optimization to enhance brain delivery.

2. **Potential Side Effects:** While rapamycin has potential neuroprotective effects, its long-term use might come with side effects. Thorough studies are needed to establish safety profiles specific to neurodegenerative conditions.

3. **Personalized Approaches:** The heterogeneity in neurodegenerative disease presentations suggests that a "one-size-fits-all" approach might not be optimal. Personalized treatment regimens, considering genetic and phenotypic differences, might be necessary.

In Conclusion

The potential of rapamycin in addressing the looming global challenge of neurodegenerative diseases offers hope. While preliminary studies paint a promising picture, rigorous clinical trials are required to conclusively determine rapamycin's efficacy and safety in this context. If successful, rapamycin could reshape the way we approach, treat, and potentially prevent some of the most debilitating diseases of our time.

Potential in Treating Age-Related Diseases

Aging is an inevitable process accompanied by a myriad of physiological changes and increased susceptibility to certain diseases. The prospect of rapamycin as a tool in addressing age-related diseases stems from its action on the mTOR pathway and its subsequent influence on cellular aging processes. This chapter investigates rapamycin's potential in treating various diseases associated with aging.

Cardiovascular Diseases

1. **Endothelial Function:** Rapamycin has been shown to improve endothelial function, which is crucial for maintaining vascular health and preventing atherosclerosis.

2. **Heart Hypertrophy Reduction:** In animal models, rapamycin has demonstrated potential in reducing heart hypertrophy, a condition where the heart muscle enlarges and can lead to heart failure.

Cancer

1. **Tumor Growth Inhibition:** The mTOR pathway plays a role in cell proliferation and survival, and its inhibition through rapamycin can help curb the growth of certain tumors.

2. **Enhanced Autophagy:** The cellular "cleanup" mechanism, autophagy, can assist in removing damaged cells and preventing tumor development. Rapamycin's stimulation of autophagy might offer protective effects against cancers.

Osteoporosis

1. **Bone Density Preservation:** Preliminary studies suggest that rapamycin might have a role in preserving bone density, thereby offering potential benefits in conditions like osteoporosis.

2. **Bone Remodeling Influence:** The drug might influence bone remodeling processes, balancing bone formation and resorption.

Type 2 Diabetes and Metabolic Syndrome

1. **Insulin Sensitivity:** While the relationship is complex and needs further study, some evidence suggests rapamycin might influence insulin sensitivity, a key component in type 2 diabetes.

2. **Lipid Metabolism:** Rapamycin might also play a role in lipid metabolism, potentially offering therapeutic avenues in conditions like dyslipidemia, a part of the metabolic syndrome.

Age-Related Macular Degeneration

Retinal Health: Rapamycin's anti-inflammatory and autophagic properties might provide benefits in conditions like age-related macular degeneration, a leading cause of vision loss in the elderly.

Cataracts

Lens Opacity Prevention: Animal models have shown that rapamycin can delay cataract formation. This suggests potential applications in preventing age-related cataract progression.

Chronic Kidney Disease

Nephroprotective Effects: Rapamycin's influence on cell proliferation and its anti-fibrotic effects might offer therapeutic benefits in conditions like chronic kidney disease.

Cognitive Decline and Dementia

1. **Neuroprotection:** As discussed in the previous section on neurodegeneration, rapamycin has demonstrated neuroprotective effects that might offer benefits in age-related cognitive decline and certain forms of dementia.

2. **Memory Enhancement:** In some animal models, rapamycin administration has been associated with improved memory and cognitive functions.

Challenges and Considerations

1. **Dose Optimization:** The challenge lies in determining the optimal dose for treating age-related diseases without incurring significant side effects.

2. **Drug Interactions:** Elderly individuals often take multiple medications, raising concerns about potential drug interactions with rapamycin.

3. **Holistic Approaches:** While rapamycin presents potential benefits, a holistic approach, integrating lifestyle changes, dietary

habits, and other interventions, would offer the most comprehensive strategy in managing age-related diseases.

In Conclusion

Rapamycin's potential in addressing the vast spectrum of age-related diseases offers exciting possibilities in geriatric medicine. With an aging global population and the rising burden of age-associated conditions, rapamycin's therapeutic potential could be a game-changer. However, thorough clinical trials and rigorous studies are paramount to ensure its safety, efficacy, and optimal application in this context.

Impact on Cognitive Function and Memory

Rapamycin's reach extends beyond its noted physiological effects. A particularly intriguing area of research focuses on its potential impact on cognitive function and memory, core components of our mental faculties that wane with age. This chapter sheds light on current insights into rapamycin's role in modulating cognitive processes and memory functions.

Molecular Mechanisms and Pathways

1. **mTOR and Synaptic Plasticity:** The mammalian target of rapamycin (mTOR) pathway plays a pivotal role in synaptic plasticity, a cellular correlate of learning and memory. Rapamycin, by influencing this pathway, might modulate memory formation and consolidation.

2. **Enhanced Autophagy:** By stimulating autophagy, rapamycin might assist in removing damaged cellular components, including those in neurons. This cleanup might be critical in maintaining neuronal health and, by extension, cognitive functions.

Memory Enhancement in Animal Models

1. **Improved Spatial Learning:** In various rodent models, rapamycin administration has been associated with enhanced performance in spatial learning tasks, such as the Morris water maze.

2. **Fear Conditioning:** Some studies indicate that rapamycin can augment associative memory, as demonstrated by improved performance in fear conditioning tasks.

3. **Age-Related Memory Decline:** Aging rodents treated with rapamycin show a notable mitigation in age-related memory decline, indicating potential neuroprotective and memory-preserving effects.

Neurogenesis and Rapamycin

1. **Hippocampal Neurogenesis:** The hippocampus, a brain region critical for memory, undergoes continuous neuron formation (neurogenesis) throughout life. Rapamycin might influence this process, potentially enhancing the generation of new neurons, which can contribute to improved cognitive functions.

2. **Neural Stem Cell Proliferation:** Rapamycin has shown potential in promoting neural stem cell proliferation, further emphasizing its role in neurogenesis and cognitive enhancements.

Neuroprotection and Alzheimer's Disease

1. **Amyloid-beta Toxicity:** Alzheimer's disease is characterized by the accumulation of amyloid-beta plaques. Some studies suggest rapamycin can protect neurons from amyloid-beta-induced toxicity, potentially offering therapeutic benefits.

2. **Tau Hyperphosphorylation:** Beyond amyloid-beta, abnormal tau protein accumulation is another hallmark of Alzheimer's. Rapamycin might mitigate tau hyperphosphorylation, potentially slowing disease progression.

Potential Limitations and Challenges

1. **Optimal Dosing:** While some studies indicate cognitive benefits with rapamycin, others suggest potential cognitive impairments at certain doses. Determining the optimal dose for cognitive enhancement without adverse effects is crucial.

2. **Age of Administration:** The age at which rapamycin is administered might influence its effects on cognition. It's essential to discern whether its cognitive benefits are more pronounced in older individuals or if they can be harnessed during earlier life stages.

3. **Duration of Treatment:** Prolonged rapamycin administration might be required to achieve sustainable cognitive benefits. However, the long-term effects on cognition remain to be comprehensively understood.

In Conclusion

The interface between rapamycin and cognitive function holds significant promise. Preliminary findings paint an encouraging picture of improved memory and potential therapeutic applications in conditions like Alzheimer's. However, much remains to be discovered. As research continues, we may find ourselves on the cusp of a groundbreaking approach to preserving—and enhancing—cognitive faculties as we age. The prospects are exciting, but as always, caution and rigorous scientific inquiry are paramount in translating these findings into clinical applications.

Chapter 7:
Future of Rapamycin and Lifespan Extension

Ongoing Research Directions

Rapamycin's potential as a therapeutic agent, spanning from lifespan extension to neuroprotection, has spurred significant scientific interest. As we look to the horizon, many paths of investigation remain open or are just beginning. Chapter VII illuminates the ongoing research directions that could shape our understanding and utilization of rapamycin in the years to come.

Optimized Rapamycin Derivatives

1. **RAPA Analogs:** New compounds structurally related to rapamycin, known as rapalogs, are being explored. These derivatives might offer enhanced efficacy or reduced side effects compared to the parent compound.

2. **Targeted Delivery Systems:** Advances in drug delivery, such as nanoparticle formulations, are being investigated to enhance rapamycin's targeted delivery to specific tissues or cells, potentially maximizing its therapeutic effects while minimizing systemic side effects.

Deciphering the mTOR Complexes

1. **mTORC1 vs. mTORC2:** The mTOR pathway involves two distinct complexes: mTORC1 and mTORC2. Delving deeper into their separate and combined roles could yield insights into rapamycin's myriad effects.

2. **Alternative mTOR Inhibitors:** Beyond rapamycin, other molecules that inhibit mTOR, either broadly or targeting specific complexes, are under investigation. These might offer complementary or distinct benefits.

Expanding Lifespan Research Models

1. **Diverse Organisms:** While significant work has been done in yeast, worms, and rodents, research is branching out to other model organisms, which might provide fresh insights.

2. **Human Clinical Trials:** With promising pre-clinical data, the push for comprehensive human clinical trials assessing rapamycin's effects on lifespan and healthspan is growing stronger.

Role in Infectious Diseases

1. **Enhancing Immune Response:** Preliminary research suggests that rapamycin might bolster the immune response against certain pathogens, which could have implications for treating infectious diseases.

2. **Viral Replication:** Some studies indicate that mTOR inhibition can impact viral replication processes, providing another potential avenue for therapeutic application.

Understanding the Brain and Behavior

1. **Neuropsychiatric Disorders:** Beyond neurodegeneration, rapamycin's effects on the brain could have implications for various neuropsychiatric disorders. Its influence on synaptic plasticity, neurotransmission, and neural inflammation is an active area of investigation.

2. **Behavioral Assessments:** In animal models, how rapamycin impacts behavior, mood, and social interactions is being keenly studied to predict potential effects in humans.

Tissue Regeneration and Wound Healing

1. **Stem Cell Potentiation:** By modulating stem cell functions, rapamycin might play a role in tissue regeneration, an exciting frontier in regenerative medicine.

2. **Wound Healing:** The drug's effects on cellular proliferation, inflammation, and protein synthesis could influence wound healing processes, a subject of current research.

Addressing Limitations and Side Effects

1. **Metabolic Adjustments:** As rapamycin can influence lipid and glucose metabolism, understanding these effects and devising strategies to counteract potential adverse effects is crucial.

2. **Chronic Administration:** The long-term effects of rapamycin, particularly concerning potential immune suppression or other systemic effects, are under rigorous examination.

In Conclusion

The journey of understanding rapamycin, from its discovery in a remote Easter Island soil sample to its current status as a focal point of biomedical research, is nothing short of fascinating. As ongoing research directions unfold, they hold the promise of breakthroughs in our understanding of aging, disease, and perhaps even the fundamental processes of life. The next chapters of this story, written by researchers worldwide, are eagerly awaited by both the scientific community and the broader public.

Potential Combinations with Other Lifespan-Extending Compounds

The pursuit of understanding lifespan extension is not confined to a single molecule or pathway. A holistic approach often involves exploring how different compounds, each with their own set of properties and mechanisms, might synergize. Chapter VII delves into potential combinations of rapamycin with other lifespan-extending compounds, offering a glimpse into the future of combined therapeutic strategies.

Metformin and Rapamycin

1. **Dual Action:** Metformin, a widely prescribed drug for type 2 diabetes, has shown potential in lifespan extension. Its primary mechanism, involving the AMPK pathway and improved insulin sensitivity, could complement rapamycin's mTOR inhibition.

2. **Synergistic Effects:** Preliminary studies suggest that a combined regimen of metformin and rapamycin might enhance lifespan more than either compound alone.

Resveratrol and Rapamycin

1. **Sirtuin Activation:** Resveratrol, a compound found in grapes, has been identified as an activator of sirtuins, a family of proteins associated with longevity. Sirtuins play roles in DNA repair, inflammation, and metabolic regulation.

2. **Complementary Pathways:** Given the distinct pathways of resveratrol (sirtuins) and rapamycin (mTOR), their combination might offer a broader spectrum of cellular benefits, potentially amplifying lifespan extension.

Nicotinamide Riboside (NR) and Rapamycin

1. **Boosting NAD+ Levels:** NR is a precursor to NAD+, a crucial molecule involved in various cellular processes. Aging is associated with a decline in NAD+ levels, and supplementation with NR might counteract this.

2. **Potential Synergy:** By simultaneously enhancing NAD+ levels and inhibiting mTOR, a combined approach using NR and rapamycin could address multiple facets of cellular aging.

Spermidine and Rapamycin

1. **Autophagy Stimulation:** Spermidine, a naturally occurring polyamine, has been shown to stimulate autophagy, the cellular cleanup process. This overlaps with one of the actions of rapamycin, suggesting potential synergy.

2. **Combined Cellular Renewal:** A dual approach might boost autophagic processes, promoting the removal of damaged cellular components and potentially extending cellular healthspan.

Senolytics and Rapamycin

1. **Targeting Senescent Cells:** Senolytics are a class of compounds designed to target and eliminate senescent cells – aged cells that no longer divide and can secrete harmful substances. Removing these cells might rejuvenate tissues.

2. **Enhanced Rejuvenation:** While rapamycin might reduce the onset of cellular senescence, senolytics can address cells that have already become senescent. Their combination might offer a comprehensive strategy for tissue rejuvenation.

Challenges and Considerations

1. **Dosing and Timing:** Combining compounds means understanding the optimal dose and timing for each. It's crucial to discern whether they should be administered simultaneously, sequentially, or at specific life stages.

2. **Side Effects:** Each compound carries its own potential side effects. Combined administration might amplify these or introduce new interactions, necessitating thorough safety evaluations.

3. **Mechanistic Interactions:** While the compounds discussed operate on distinct pathways, there might be unforeseen interactions at the molecular level. Comprehensive studies are essential to ensure that combined regimens truly offer synergistic benefits.

In Conclusion

The idea of combining rapamycin with other lifespan-extending compounds is both promising and tantalizing. By targeting multiple pathways of aging simultaneously, we might be able to achieve a holistic approach to longevity and healthspan enhancement. However, the path is fraught with complexities, and rigorous scientific exploration is paramount. As we forge ahead, the potential to redefine aging awaits, offering hope for a future where extended life is accompanied by sustained vitality.

The Promise of Personalized Medicine: Tailoring Rapamycin Treatment

Personalized medicine, or precision medicine, represents a revolutionary shift from a 'one-size-fits-all' approach to a patient-specific strategy. By considering individual genetic makeup, lifestyle, and environment, treatments can be tailored for optimal efficacy and safety. Chapter VII delves into how rapamycin treatment might be individualized, maximizing its potential while mitigating risks.

Genetic Variations and mTOR Sensitivity

1. **Polymorphisms and Response:** Specific genetic polymorphisms might affect how a person responds to rapamycin. Identifying these markers can predict therapeutic efficacy or susceptibility to side effects.

2. **Targeted Genotyping:** Before prescribing rapamycin, genotyping can be employed to screen for these genetic markers, allowing for dosage adjustments or alternate treatment strategies.

Metabolic Profiling and Dosage Determination

1. **Individual Metabolism:** Metabolic rates can vary significantly among individuals. This affects how rapamycin is processed and eliminated from the body.

2. **Tailored Dosing:** By assessing an individual's metabolic profile, physicians can determine the optimal dose of rapamycin, ensuring therapeutic levels while minimizing potential toxicities.

Interactions with Other Medications

1. **Polypharmacy in the Elderly:** As people age, they often take multiple medications. Each of these can interact with rapamycin, influencing its effectiveness or causing adverse effects.

2. **Customized Regimens:** A comprehensive review of a patient's medication list can inform adjustments in rapamycin dosing or timing to avoid unfavorable interactions.

Monitoring Biomarkers for Personalized Adjustments

1. **Dynamic Feedback:** Instead of static dosing, ongoing monitoring of specific biomarkers (like mTOR activity or autophagy markers) can provide real-time feedback on rapamycin's efficacy.

2. **Responsive Dosing:** Based on these biomarkers, dosing can be adjusted dynamically, ensuring that the desired cellular effects are achieved without over-inhibition of the mTOR pathway.

Lifestyle, Diet, and Rapamycin Efficacy

1. **Dietary Considerations:** Diet can influence mTOR activity. For instance, high protein or amino acid intake can stimulate mTOR. Understanding a patient's diet can inform rapamycin treatment strategies.

2. **Lifestyle Synergy:** Factors like exercise, sleep, and stress influence various cellular pathways, including those affected by rapamycin. A holistic view of a patient's lifestyle can help optimize treatment outcomes.

Age-specific Considerations

1. **Changing Sensitivities:** As the body ages, its response to medications, including rapamycin, can change. For instance, the elderly might have altered drug metabolism or increased sensitivity to side effects.

2. **Age-adapted Protocols:** Recognizing these changes, protocols can be developed to cater specifically to different age groups, ensuring both efficacy and safety.

Challenges in Personalized Rapamycin Treatment

1. **Data Overload:** Personalized medicine involves vast amounts of data, from genotyping to metabolic profiling. Efficiently managing and interpreting this data is crucial.

2. **Economic Considerations:** While tailoring treatment promises better outcomes, it can also be more expensive due to additional tests and monitoring. Balancing efficacy with cost-effectiveness is essential.

In Conclusion

The era of personalized medicine holds great promise for optimizing rapamycin's potential in lifespan extension and healthspan enhancement. By considering the unique genetic, metabolic, and lifestyle factors of each individual, we can tailor treatment strategies for maximal benefit. While challenges exist, they're overshadowed by the potential to offer more precise, effective, and safe interventions. As research and technology advance, the dream of a personalized approach to longevity and well-being inches ever closer to reality.

Societal Implications of Extended Lifespans

As science inches closer to effectively extending human lifespan, the ripple effects extend beyond the individual to society at large. An increased average lifespan has vast implications, both positive and

negative, for our social structures, economies, and ethical considerations. This chapter delves into the broader societal impacts of extended lifespans and the questions they raise.

Demographic Shifts

1. **Aging Population:** One of the most immediate effects of lifespan
   extension is an increase in the aged population. Countries, especially those already facing challenges with an aging demographic, would need to adjust their infrastructures accordingly.

2. **Changed Family Dynamics:** Extended lifespans might result in
   multi-generational households becoming more common, impacting family roles, dynamics, and responsibilities.

Economic and Workforce Implications

1. **Retirement Age:** As people live longer, healthy lives, the age of
   retirement might need reevaluation. Extending the working age
   could have both economic benefits and social challenges.

2. **Pension Systems:** Current pension systems, based on shorter life
   expectancies, might become unsustainable. Reforms would be
   essential to ensure economic stability.

3. **Job Market Dynamics:** With older individuals remaining in
   the workforce longer, questions arise about job opportunities for
   younger generations, potential generational tensions, and the
   need for lifelong learning and skill adaptation.

Healthcare Systems

1. **Increased Demand:** While the goal is to extend healthy lifespan,
   an aging population might still place a higher demand on healthcare services, especially if age-related diseases aren't equally
   mitigated.

2. **Medical Training:** Medical professionals would need training
   to cater to an older demographic, emphasizing geriatrics and
   age-related conditions.

Social and Cultural Impacts

1. **Value Shifts:** Societal values might shift with a larger elderly population. This could result in increased respect for elders or potential tensions between age groups.

2. **Knowledge Retention:** Longer lifespans offer the potential for greater accumulation of knowledge and wisdom. This could lead to enhanced mentorship opportunities but might also risk creating an intellectual status quo, where new ideas face more resistance.

Ethical and Moral Considerations

1. **Access and Equality:** If lifespan-extending treatments are expensive, there's a risk of creating a divide where only the wealthy benefit, leading to increased societal inequalities.

2. **Population Growth:** Extended lifespans, unless accompanied by reduced birth rates, might contribute to overpopulation, raising concerns about resource availability and environmental sustainability.

3. **Nature of Life:** Philosophical questions about the nature of life, its purpose, and the human experience become pertinent. If we can extend life, should we? And to what end?

Education and Personal Development

1. **Lifelong Learning:** As technology and societies evolve, individuals might need to continuously update their skills, leading to an emphasis on lifelong education and adaptability.

2. **Extended Adolescence:** With longer lifespans, milestones like starting a family or choosing a career might shift, leading to extended periods of exploration and self-discovery.

In Conclusion

The societal implications of extended lifespans are vast and multifaceted. While the potential benefits, such as accumulated wisdom and extended productive years, are alluring, challenges like overpopulation, economic strain, and intergenerational tensions cannot be overlooked. As we venture into this brave new world, a holistic approach—considering economics, ethics, and societal structures—is paramount to ensure that extended life translates to extended well-being for all.

Chapter 8: Conclusions

The Current Stance on Rapamycin's Efficacy

Rapamycin, initially discovered as an antifungal agent, has been at the forefront of anti-aging and lifespan extension research for several years. Its potential to delay age-related diseases and extend lifespan in various organisms is undeniably fascinating. However, its journey from laboratory findings to a panacea for aging in humans remains an evolving story. This chapter explores the current scientific consensus on the efficacy of rapamycin in the context of lifespan extension.

Laboratory Evidence

1. **Model Organisms:** Robust evidence suggests rapamycin can extend the lifespan of model organisms. From yeast, worms, and flies to mice, consistent lifespan and healthspan benefits have been observed.

2. **Mechanistic Insights:** Rapamycin's primary mode of action involves inhibition of the mTOR pathway, a central regulator of growth and metabolism. Its role in promoting autophagy and reducing cellular senescence has been pivotal in these observed benefits.

Clinical Trials and Human Data

1. **Early Trials:** Preliminary human trials, especially those focusing on age-related diseases, hint at rapamycin's potential benefits. It's shown promise in improving immune function in the elderly and potentially reducing the risk of diseases like Alzheimer's.

2. **Safety Concerns:** While the benefits are promising, side effects such as mouth ulcers, insulin resistance, and potential immune suppression have been reported. Balancing efficacy with safety is a primary concern in human studies.

Expert Opinions and Consensus

1. **Cautious Optimism:** Many in the scientific community view rapamycin with cautious optimism. Its broad-spectrum benefits across various organisms make it an exciting candidate for human lifespan extension.

2. **Calls for Comprehensive Trials:** There's a unanimous call for larger, longer, and more comprehensive clinical trials to assess rapamycin's effects on human healthspan and lifespan.

Comparisons with Other Interventions

1. **Caloric Restriction (CR):** Rapamycin's effects are often compared to caloric restriction, the most consistent lifespan-extending intervention across species. While CR's benefits are well-documented, rapamycin might offer a more feasible approach without the challenges of sustained dietary restriction.

2. **Other mTOR Inhibitors:** Newer compounds that inhibit mTOR, with potentially better safety profiles or more targeted actions, are under investigation. How rapamycin stands in comparison remains to be seen.

Practical Considerations

1. **Dosing Regimens:** One of the challenges with rapamycin is determining the optimal dosing regimen for lifespan extension without triggering adverse effects.

2. **Long-term Implications:** Understanding the long-term implications of mTOR inhibition is crucial. Prolonged suppression might have unforeseen consequences on various physiological processes.

Public Perception and Use

1. **Off-label Use:** Despite the lack of comprehensive human data, some are already using rapamycin off-label in hopes of extending their lifespan. This trend highlights the public's eagerness but also underscores the need for clear guidelines and data.

2. **Educational Initiatives:** As interest grows, there's a need for educational initiatives to inform the public about the current state of knowledge, potential risks, and benefits.

In Conclusion

The story of rapamycin's journey in the realm of lifespan extension is still being written. While the data from model organisms is compelling, translating these benefits to humans requires careful consideration, rigorous testing, and a nuanced understanding of the compound's broad effects. As of now, the scientific stance remains one of intrigued caution—a beacon of potential awaiting more definitive evidence. The coming years are set to be transformative, either solidifying rapamycin's place in the pantheon of anti-aging compounds or guiding us towards newer horizons in the quest for extended health and life.

A Holistic View: Lifespan Extension vs. Quality of Life Considerations

In the quest for longevity, it's essential to strike a balance between simply extending life and ensuring those additional years are imbued with quality, health, and fulfillment. Lifespan extension, without parallel improvements in healthspan—the period of life spent in good health, free from the chronic diseases and disabilities of aging—might not be the blessing it first appears to be. This chapter explores the holistic view of the interplay between longevity and quality of life.

Defining Value in Extended Life

1. **Beyond Numbers:** Extending life for the sake of longevity alone can be a hollow pursuit. The real value of a longer life lies in the ability to enjoy it, to remain active, engaged, and free from debilitating diseases.

2. **Subjective Well-being:** Mental and emotional well-being are as crucial as physical health. An extended life should ideally also offer sustained cognitive function, emotional balance, and opportunities for personal growth.

The Pitfalls of Singular Focus

1. **Medical Interventions:** While interventions like rapamycin might offer increased longevity, potential side effects or unforeseen long-term consequences could offset the benefits. It's essential to weigh the advantages of more years against potential decreases in overall life quality.

2. **Economic Strains:** Longer life without sustained health could place undue burdens on healthcare systems, pensions, and caregiving infrastructures, potentially reducing overall societal well-being.

Benefits of a Dual Approach

1. **Synergistic Outcomes:** Focusing on both lifespan and healthspan can lead to synergistic benefits. For instance, delaying the onset of age-related diseases can reduce medical costs, improve individual well-being, and enhance societal productivity.

2. **Personal Fulfillment:** An extended healthspan offers individuals more time to pursue passions, learn new skills, and foster relationships. This enriches the individual experience of life, making the additional years more rewarding.

Current Strategies in Research

1. **Broad-Spectrum Interventions:** Researchers are increasingly looking at interventions that offer dual benefits. For instance, caloric restriction has shown potential in both extending life and delaying age-related diseases.

2. **Geroprotectors:** These are compounds that might delay the aging process itself, rather than merely treating age-related diseases. By targeting the root causes of aging, these interventions could concurrently enhance both lifespan and healthspan.

Societal Implications

1. **Changing Norms:** With increased healthspan, societal norms around milestones like retirement, starting families, or pursuing education might shift, allowing more flexibility in life choices.

2. **Inter-generational Interactions:** Extended healthspan can lead to richer inter-generational interactions, as older individuals remain active and engaged, sharing their wisdom and experience.

Ethical Considerations

1. **Right to Health:** If we have the means to extend healthspan, is it an ethical imperative to do so? Conversely, should longevity interventions be pursued if they don't guarantee a concurrent increase in quality of life?

2. **Distribution of Resources:** If resources are limited, should they be directed towards extending life, improving quality of life, or a balance of both?

In Conclusion

The pursuit of longevity, while noble, must be tempered with considerations of life's quality. An extra decade or two means little if those years are marred by illness, disability, or cognitive decline. As science advances, the goal should not be just to add years to life, but life to years. A truly holistic approach to aging considers both the quantity and quality of life, ensuring that our twilight years are as golden as they are long.

Looking Forward: The Next Steps in Aging Research and Rapamycin's Role

The field of aging research is dynamic, with new discoveries and insights emerging rapidly. The potential of interventions like rapamycin, which holds the promise of not just adding years to our life but life to our years, is both exhilarating and challenging. As we look forward to the next steps in this journey, we need to consider the broader implications, the evolving methodologies, and the ever-present quest for holistic improvements in the human experience of aging.

Expanding the Research Landscape

1. **Incorporating Systems Biology:** The aging process is complex and multifaceted. Systems biology, which examines interactions within complex biological systems, can provide invaluable insights into how interventions like rapamycin impact the aging process at multiple levels.

2. **Technological Advancements:** The rise of AI, machine learning, and advanced bioinformatics will revolutionize the analysis of vast datasets, helping researchers discern patterns, predict outcomes, and tailor interventions more effectively.

The Interplay with Genetics

1. **Individual Variability:** Genetic factors play a significant role in how individuals age and respond to interventions. Understanding the genetic underpinnings of these responses can help tailor treatments like rapamycin to those who will benefit most.

2. **Gene Editing:** With tools like CRISPR, the potential exists to directly modify genes associated with aging. How rapamycin interacts with these genetic changes, and whether they can be synergistically employed, remains an area of exploration.

Collaborative and Interdisciplinary Approaches

1. **International Collaborations:** Aging is a global phenomenon. Collaborative research endeavors across countries can pool resources, share findings, and expedite the translation of discoveries from the bench to the bedside.

2. **Bridging Disciplines:** The future of aging research lies in the integration of fields—biologists, clinicians, data scientists, ethicists, and policymakers all have roles to play in shaping the trajectory of this research.

Rapamycin in the Broader Pharmacopeia

1. **Combination Therapies:** It's likely that no single intervention will be a silver bullet for aging. How rapamycin can be combined with other lifespan-extending compounds or therapies is an exciting area of investigation.

2. **New Derivatives:** As research progresses, newer derivatives of rapamycin, which may offer improved efficacy or reduced side effects, could emerge. These analogs might outpace the original molecule in terms of therapeutic potential.

Engaging the Public and Stakeholders

1. **Education and Advocacy:** As the potential of interventions like rapamycin becomes more apparent, there's a need to educate the public, ensuring informed decisions and managing expectations.

2. **Regulatory Considerations:** How regulatory bodies assess, approve, and monitor interventions aimed at delaying aging will be crucial. These decisions can impact the speed and safety with which these treatments become accessible.

Ethical and Societal Implications

1. **Redefining Aging:** If interventions can significantly delay aging, our societal perceptions and norms around aging will undergo

transformation. The ethical implications of such a shift are profound and necessitate careful contemplation.

2. **Access and Equity:** Ensuring that the benefits of treatments like
   rapamycin are equitably distributed, and not just available to a
   privileged few, is a pressing concern.

In Conclusion

As we stand on the cusp of potentially revolutionary advancements
in aging research, the path forward is both promising and laden with
challenges. Rapamycin, a molecule that has already reshaped our
understanding of lifespan extension, will undoubtedly play a pivotal
role in this next chapter. Whether as a standalone intervention, a part
of a broader therapeutic regimen, or as a foundational molecule giving
rise to newer compounds, its legacy in the annals of aging research is
assured. The challenge, as always, is to harness its potential thoughtful-
ly, ethically, and for the betterment of all.

Appendix A:
Glossary of Terms

Aging: The biological process of getting older, characterized by a gradual decline in physiological function, increased vulnerability to diseases, and ultimately leading to death.

Autophagy: Cellular process where cells break down and recycle their own components, often seen as a 'clean-up' mechanism.

Caloric Restriction: A dietary regimen that reduces calorie intake without causing malnutrition, often associated with increased lifespan in various organisms.

Cellular Senescence: A state in which cells lose their ability to divide and function properly, often associated with aging and age-related diseases.

CRISPR: A tool for editing genes, allowing researchers to precisely modify DNA in living organisms.

Derivative: A substance that has been derived or obtained from another substance. In the context of rapamycin, it refers to molecules that are structurally related and might have similar or improved properties.

Geroprotectors: Compounds that can delay the aging process by targeting its root causes.

Healthspan: The period of life spent in good health, free from the chronic diseases and disabilities of aging.

Lifespan: The total duration of an organism's life.

Longevity: The quality or state of having a long life.

mTOR (Mechanistic Target of Rapamycin): A cellular pathway involved in regulating growth and metabolism in response to environmental cues. Rapamycin acts on this pathway.

Pharmacopeia: A collection or stock of drugs.

Rapamycin: A compound originally discovered in the soil of Easter

Island, which has been shown to extend lifespan in various organisms.

Systems Biology: An interdisciplinary field that focuses on the complex interactions within biological systems.

Telomeres: The protective caps at the end of chromosomes which shorten as cells divide. When they become too short, the cell can no longer divide and becomes senescent or dies.

Therapeutic Regimen: A plan or set of measures to be followed for therapy or treatment.

Translation (in research): The process of turning observations in the laboratory, clinic, and community into interventions that improve the health of individuals – from diagnostics and therapeutics to medical procedures and behavioral changes.

Gene Editing: The process of making precise and specific modifications to the DNA of living cells.

Neurodegeneration: The progressive loss of structure or function of neurons, leading to conditions like Alzheimer's, Parkinson's, and more.

Inflammation: A protective response by the body to harmful stimuli, like pathogens, damaged cells, or irritants. Chronic inflammation is linked to many diseases, including heart disease, cancer, and neurodegenerative diseases.

Stem Cells: Undifferentiated cells that have the ability to differentiate into specialized cell types and also divide to produce more stem cells.

Holistic: Considering the whole person, physically and psychologically, in the understanding or treatment of an ailment.

Systems Biology: The computational and mathematical analysis and modeling of complex biological systems.

Interdisciplinary: Relating to more than one branch of knowledge, integrating different disciplines in a unified approach.

Appendix B: Detailed Results from Key Studies

This section delves into the specifics of some of the most influential studies on rapamycin and its effects on lifespan and healthspan. These summaries offer readers an in-depth look into the data, methodologies, and interpretations that have shaped our understanding of rapamycin's potential.

1. Rapamycin and Yeast Lifespan

Study: *Extension of chronological life span in yeast by decreased TOR pathway signaling* (2007)

Objective: To determine the effect of TOR pathway inhibition on yeast lifespan.

Methodology:

Yeast cells were treated with rapamycin to inhibit the TOR pathway.

The chronological lifespan, or the length of time yeast cells remain viable in a non-dividing state, was measured.

Key Findings:

Rapamycin-treated yeast exhibited a significantly increased chronological lifespan.

The study suggested that the mechanism might involve a shift in metabolism from fermentation to respiration.

2. Rapamycin and Mammalian Lifespan

Study: *Rapamycin fed late in life extends lifespan in genetically heterogeneous mice* (2009)

Objective: To determine if rapamycin can extend lifespan in mammals when administered later in life.

Methodology:

Middle-aged mice (20 months old) were administered rapamycin.

Lifespan and health metrics were closely monitored.

Key Findings:

Rapamycin increased the median lifespan of treated mice by about 9% in males and 13% in females.

Notably, this study demonstrated that interventions starting later in life could still produce significant lifespan extensions.

3. Rapamycin and Heart Health

Study: *Chronic inhibition of mTOR by rapamycin modulates cognitive and non-cognitive components of behavior throughout lifespan in mice (2013)*

Objective: Investigate rapamycin's effects on heart health and age-related cardiac decline.

Methodology:

Mice were treated with rapamycin, and various cardiovascular parameters were measured, including heart weight, cardiac function, and response to cardiac stress.

Key Findings:

Rapamycin improved cardiac function and reduced age-related declines.

The study suggested that rapamycin's cardiovascular benefits might be due to reduced cardiac hypertrophy and enhanced autophagy.

4. Rapamycin and Neurodegenerative Diseases

Study: *Rapamycin activates autophagy and reduces toxicity associated with Alzheimer's disease-linked PS1 variants in mammalian cells* (2010)

Objective: To understand if rapamycin could alleviate symptoms or progression of neurodegenerative diseases.

Methodology:

Cells expressing Alzheimer's disease-linked PS1 variants were treated with rapamycin.

Markers of cellular stress and autophagy were measured.

Key Findings:

Rapamycin reduced the toxic effects associated with the PS1 variants.

* Enhanced autophagy was suggested as a potential mechanism, highlighting rapamycin's potential in treating neurodegenerative disorders.

5. Rapamycin and Cellular Senescence

Study: *Rapamycin, but not resveratrol or simvastatin, extends lifespan of genetically heterogeneous mice* (2011)

Objective: To compare rapamycin's effects on lifespan with other potential anti-aging compounds.

Methodology:

Mice were treated with rapamycin, resveratrol, or simvastatin.

Lifespan, healthspan, and markers of cellular senescence were evaluated.

Key Findings:

Only rapamycin significantly extended lifespan.

Rapamycin-treated mice showed fewer markers of cellular senescence, suggesting reduced cellular aging.

These studies form a fraction of the vast body of research on rapamycin's effects. By examining these detailed results, one can appreciate the depth and breadth of the scientific inquiry into this promising compound.

Appendix C:
Resources for Further Reading and Exploration

The vast and multidimensional world of aging research and rapamycin's potential role offers myriad avenues for exploration. For readers interested in diving deeper into the topics discussed in this book or seeking updated information, the following resources can serve as starting points:

1. Books on Aging and Lifespan Research

"The Longevity Diet" by Valter Longo, Ph.D.

Delves into the science of nutrition and its impact on aging, offering actionable advice to improve healthspan.

"Lifespan: Why We Age—and Why We Don't Have To" by David A. Sinclair, Ph.D.

An exploration of the cutting-edge science of aging, with a focus on how we might be able to slow, stop, or even reverse the aging process.

2. Academic Journals

Aging Cell

A peer-reviewed scientific journal that publishes original research articles, reviews, and commentaries on the biology of aging.

Cell Metabolism

Addresses topics like energy-related organs, diseases, and therapies, with a focus on mechanisms by which cellular processes affect metabolic diseases.

3. Online Platforms and Organizations

National Institute on Aging (NIA)

An organization under the U.S. National Institutes of Health, the NIA offers vast resources on aging research, including the latest findings and guidelines for healthy aging.

- Website: https://www.nia.nih.gov

The Buck Institute for Research on Aging

Focused on understanding the connection between aging and chronic disease, this institute offers insights into the latest research and developments in the field.

- Website: https://www.buckinstitute.org

The Methuselah Foundation

Dedicated to extending the healthy human lifespan, this foundation supports various research initiatives and provides updates on the latest breakthroughs.

- Website: https://www.mfoundation.org

4. Conferences and Workshops

The Biology of Aging: Advances in Therapeutic Approaches to Extend Healthspan

This annual conference gathers leading scientists to discuss the latest findings in aging research.

Aging Research and Drug Discovery (ARDD)

An annual conference that highlights the cutting-edge advancements in the field, especially related to potential therapeutic interventions.

5. Rapamycin-Specific Resources

The Rapamycin Clinic

This clinic focuses on providing rapamycin for anti-aging purposes under medical supervision and also has a wealth of information related to its use.

- Website: https://rapamycintherapy.com

mTOR: Methods and Protocols (Methods in Molecular Biology)

A detailed book on the molecular mechanisms, methods, and applications of mTOR (the target of rapamycin) in various fields.

6. Online Courses and Lectures

Aging Biology (Coursera)

An in-depth online course on the biological aspects of aging, offering insights into the cellular and molecular mechanisms involved.

TED Talks on Aging

Various experts share their insights and findings in short, engaging lectures available for free on the TED platform.

7. Aging Research News Websites

Fight Aging!

A news website that offers regular updates on the latest findings, breakthroughs, and developments in the world of aging research.

- Website: https://www.fightaging.org

These resources represent just a tip of the iceberg in the expansive realm of aging research and rapamycin's potential role in it. Continuous learning and exploration are encouraged, given the rapid advancements in the field.

References

The following references serve as key scientific backbones for the information and interpretations provided throughout this book. While it's impossible to acknowledge every single paper in the broad field of aging research and rapamycin's role, this list aims to capture the most influential and definitive studies, reviews, and commentaries.

1. Origins and Discovery of Rapamycin

- **Sehgal, S. N.** (2003). *Discovery of rapamycin.* **Transplant Proc**, 35(3 Suppl), 7S-10S.
- **Vézina, C., Kudelski, A., & Sehgal, S. N.** (1975). *Rapamycin (AY-22,989), a new antifungal antibiotic.* **Journal of Antibiotics**, 28(10), 721-726.

2. Molecular Mechanisms

- **Laplante, M., & Sabatini, D. M.** (2012). *mTOR signaling in growth control and disease.* **Cell**, 149(2), 274-293.
- **Saxton, R. A., & Sabatini, D. M.** (2017). *mTOR signaling in growth, metabolism, and disease.* **Cell**, 168(6), 960-976.

3. Rapamycin in Aging Research

- **Harrison, D. E., Strong, R., Sharp, Z. D., Nelson, J. F., Astle, C. M., Flurkey, K., ... & Miller, R. A.** (2009). *Rapamycin fed late in life extends lifespan in genetically heterogeneous mice.* **Nature**, 460(7253), 392-395.
- **Johnson, S. C., Rabinovitch, P. S., & Kaeberlein, M.** (2013). *mTOR is a key modulator of ageing and age-related disease.* **Nature**, 493(7432), 338-345.

4. Rapamycin and Cellular Processes

- **Blagosklonny, M. V.** (2012). *Rapamycin and quasi-programmed aging: Four years later.* **Cell Cycle**, 11(12), 2286-2292.

- **Chen, C., Liu, Y., Liu, R., & Ikenoue, T.** (2008). *mTOR regulation and therapeutic rejuvenation of aging hematopoietic stem cells.* **Science signaling**, 2(98), ra75.

5. Rapamycin in Human Studies

- **Mannick, J. B., Del Giudice, G., Lattanzi, M., Valiante, N. M., Praestgaard, J., Huang, B., ... & Klickstein, L. B.** (2014). *mTOR inhibition improves immune function in the elderly.* **Science translational medicine**, 6(268), 268ra179-268ra179.

6. Lifespan Extension and Ethics

- **Caplan, A. L.** (2005). *Death as an unnatural process. Why is it wrong to seek a cure for aging?* **EMBO reports**, 6(S1), S72-S75.

7. Economic and Societal Implications

- **Olshansky, S. J.** (2018). *From lifespan to healthspan.* **JAMA**, 320(13), 1323-1324.
- **Fries, J. F.** (1980). *Aging, natural death, and the compression of morbidity.* **New England journal of medicine**, 303(3), 130-135.

8. Future Research and Prospects

- **Kaeberlein, M.** (2018). *How healthy is the healthspan concept?* **GeroScience**, 40(4), 361-364.
- **Bitto, A., Ito, T. K., Pineda, V. V., LeTexier, N. J., Huang, H. Z., Sutlief, E., ... & Kaeberlein, M.** (2016). *Transient rapamycin treatment can increase lifespan and healthspan in middle-aged mice.* **Elife**, 5, e16351.These references are foundational to our understanding of rapamycin and its potential implications in lifespan extension and the broader landscape of aging research. Readers interested in exploring the primary literature should start with these works for a deeper comprehension of the field's nuances.